# THE SHOCKING REALITY OF
# VIOLENCE IN HEALTHCARE

## AND WHAT WE CAN DO ABOUT IT

Sheila Wilson, RN, BSN, MPH

*Edited by Jamie L. Ross*

# COPYRIGHT

# TABLE OF CONTENTS

# INTRODUCTION

I have worked as a nurse for over four decades. Over the course of that time, I have witnessed and been a victim of workplace violence.

By 2008, I and some of my colleagues realized something had to be done to stop assault against healthcare workers.

In 2009, I co-founded the organization Stop Healthcare Violence, with the mission to educate and inform the public on the alarming epidemic of violence committed against healthcare personnel, provide support and advocacy for victims, and lobby for legislative change.

As an extension of this organization's goals, I wrote this book to help my fellow nursing colleagues identify potentially dangerous situations, protect themselves, diminish incidents of healthcare violence, and understand something very important: *being a victim of assault is not acceptable, and it is not within your job description.*

Did you get that?

*Being a victim of assault is not acceptable, and it is not within your job description.*

It never was.

If you feel that it is part of your nursing responsibilities, please read that job description again.

**Imagine this scenario...**

*You are Sally, a bank loan officer, discussing mortgage refinancing with Blake, your applicant. Displeased with the information you give him, Blake becomes enraged and spits in your face, curses viciously, and hurls a stapler at you.*

Would this be okay?

Would you accept the incident, brush it aside, never reporting to security staff, bank management, local police?

Of course not.

Whether the stapler struck you in the face, grazed your arm, or missed you entirely, the answer would be *no*.

*No,* this would not be okay; *no,* you would never brush it aside; and *no,* your employer would never expect you to.

Yet nurses and healthcare workers are being assaulted on an ongoing and escalating basis, and only a few are identifying it as violence and treating it as wrong, criminal and stoppable.

In fact, a 2015 article in The Permanente Journal cited:

> *...workplace violence is increasing across the nation's Emergency Departments (EDs) and nurses often perceive it as part of their job.*

Well, guess what? Workplace violence *is, indeed, increasing, not only in the ED, but in all aspects of nursing,* and *it's not part of any job.*

Whether you have been a victim of healthcare violence, know someone who has, or simply wish to put an end to this epidemic, read on; this book is for you.

Sheila Wilson, RN, BSN, MPH
Co-Founder and President
Stop Healthcare Violence
www.StopHealthcareViolence.org

---

[1] www.tinyurl.com/permanente-journal

## PART I

# WHAT'S ALL THE FUSS ABOUT?

## THE MANY STRATA OF HEALTHCARE VIOLENCE

# WHAT IS WORKPLACE VIOLENCE?

Before we can talk about *healthcare violence*, we have to back up a step, and briefly relate on the broader spectrum of *workplace violence.*

According to the U.S. Department of Occupational Safety and Health Administration (OSHA)[2]:

> *Workplace violence (WPV) is any act or threat of physical violence, harassment, intimidation, or other threatening disruptive behavior that occurs at the work site. It ranges from threats and verbal abuse to physical assaults and even homicide. It can affect and involve employees, clients, customers and visitors… However it manifests itself, workplace violence is a major concern for employers and employees nationwide.*

Let me be clear: workplace violence is not simplistic, nor is it isolated. Workplace violence is complicated, and it is rampant. Workplace violence isn't simply a matter of being hit, verbally assaulted, spit upon or pushed, and then forgetting about it, moving along. Like an onion, workplace violence itself involves many layers, as do the elements and strata that

---

[2] www.tinyurl.com/osha-wpv-overview

contribute to this ever-increasing pandemic and enable its existence.

And also like an onion, workplace violence can bring tears to your eyes - in more ways than one.

# VIOLENCE IN HEALTHCARE

## Healthcare Violence: An Epidemic All its Own

According to OSHA, workplace violence poses a specifically grave threat in the healthcare industry:

> *Workers in hospitals, nursing homes, and other healthcare settings face significant risks of workplace violence. Many factors contribute to this risk, including working directly with people who have a history of violence or who may be delirious or under the influence of drugs. From 2002 to 2013, the rate of serious workplace violence incidents (those requiring days off for an injured worker to recuperate) was more than four times greater in healthcare than in private industry on average. In fact, healthcare accounts for nearly as many serious violent injuries as all other industries combined. Many more assaults or threats go unreported.*

The Emergency Nurses Association[3] echoes this viewpoint:

> *It is the position of the Emergency Nurses Association that Emergency nurses are at significant occupational risk for WPV.*

---

[3] www.tinyurl.com/ena-violence-in-er

As does the American Nurses Association[4]:

*Workplace violence is one of the most complex and dangerous occupational hazards facing nurses working in today's health care environment.*

And the APNA[5]:

*The American Psychiatric Nurses Association (APNA), the largest professional organization for psychiatric nurses, recognizes that violence in the workplace is a pressing occupational concern...*

And last but not least, OSHA's Guidelines for Preventing Workplace Violence[6] states:

*Healthcare and social service workers face a significant risk of job-related violence. The National Institute for Occupational Safety and Health (NIOSH) defines workplace violence as "violent acts (including physical assaults and threats of assaults) directed toward persons at work or on duty." According to the Bureau of Labor Statistics (BLS), 27 out of the 100 fatalities in healthcare and social service settings that occurred in 2013 were due to assaults and violent acts.*

---

[4] www.tinyurl.com/ana-wpv-in-healthcare
[5] www.tinyurl.com/apna-position-statement
[6] www.tinyurl.com/osha-guidelines

My career as a nurse spans more than 40 years. Over that time I have witnessed and experienced violence.

The concept of violence against healthcare workers is unfathomably wrong on so many levels. Shouldn't we feel safe, and be safe, from violent threats and physical harm in the workplace? Isn't it, in fact, our legal right, under Federal law[7], *to be safe from harm in the workplace?* (By the way and spoiler alert: You will encounter this message several times within this book, just to drive the point home.)

[7] www.osha.gov/workers/index.html

# WHO IS AT RISK?

For many of us – in fact, for most of us – everyday life can be difficult at times. Yet for my healthcare colleagues, those life difficulties are greatly compounded simply by going to work every day. Countless numbers of healthcare workers, near and far, have left for work one day just like any other day and returned home with a completely altered existence.

It should be noted that those at risk are not limited to hospital staff. OSHA[8] points out that at-risk settings also include:

- **Residential Treatment** settings, including institutional facilities such as nursing homes, and other long-term care facilities

- **Non-residential Treatment/Service** settings including small neighborhood clinics and mental health centers

- **Community Care** settings including community-based residential facilities and group homes

- **Field work** settings including home healthcare workers or social workers who make home visits

---

[8] www.tinyurl.com/osha-guidelines

# THE STATS SPEAK

A 2011 study by the Emergency Nurses Association found that 54% of ER nurses reported having experienced physical violence and/or verbal abuse from a patient and/or visitor during the previous seven calendar days.

Did you catch that? *More than half* of ER nurses, in a calendar week, were assaulted.

Keep in mind:

- Underreporting (failing to report) incidents of healthcare violence are actually skewing the statistics to appear more conservative than they actually are.

- These statistics are from 2011 - *five years prior to this book's original publication* - and that the numbers reflect attacks on ER staff *only*. Patients, if admitted, go to the floor, where assaults on unit staff also occur. In fact, studies have shown that between 35% and 80% of hospital staff has been physically assaulted at least once during their careers, and 46% of all non-fatal assaults and violent acts requiring days away from work were

---

[9] www.tinyurl.com/ena-study
[10] www.tinyurl.com/ena-toolkit

committed against registered nurses. Consider these more recent findings from the Bureau of Labor Statistics:

*In a 2014 survey[11], almost 80 percent of nurses reported being attacked on the job within the past year. Health-care workers experience the most nonfatal workplace violence compared to other professions by a wide margin, with attacks on them accounting for almost 70 percent of all nonfatal workplace assaults causing days away from work in the U.S.*

Healthcare workers are often verbally abused, cursed at, threatened, hit, slapped, shoved, bitten, and have objects thrown at them.

And patients are not the sole perpetrators of healthcare violence, either, as illustrated by OSHA[12]:

*In hospitals, nursing homes, and other healthcare settings, possible sources of violence include patients, visitors, intruders, and even coworkers. Examples include verbal threats or physical attacks by patients, a distraught family member who may be abusive or even become an active shooter, gang violence in the emergency department, a domestic dispute that spills over into the workplace, or coworker bullying.*

---

[11] www.tinyurl.com/journal-emergency-nursing
[12] www.tinyurl.com/osha-wpv-in-healthcare

So when someone ponders, "Is the violence really that bad?"

The answer is *yes*.

Consider this from a writer for Nurse.com[13]:

> *As healthcare workers, we never know whether we will return home in the same condition in which we started work - or even whether we will return home at all.*

---

[13] www.tinyurl.com/nurse-danger-zone

## A LIFE CHANGED IN A HEARTBEAT

Episodes of assault leave physical scars, permanent ailments, and emotional trauma. Rarely, if ever, does an assault victim walk away completely unscathed. For these victims, life is changed in a heartbeat.

I have heard people say, "Oh, come on; did you get really hurt? You work in a hospital, for goodness sake - people come in and hurt you? Now, really, how can that possibly be true?"

*Yes*, I think. *I feel the same way: how can this possibly be true?*

Or I've been asked, "Did that patient's bite really hurt you so badly?"

*Yes, it did hurt that badly, and afterward, I was out of work for four days and required a prescription antibiotic because my finger became infected.*

To me and to some of my colleagues, this reality feels like a parallel universe, a sentiment expressed by one coworker who'd been a victim of assault:

> *I went into nursing to help people, not to get hurt and be threatened.*

Jeff, another ER nurse, echoes:

> *You sign up for this job thinking you're going to help people,*
> *and then you have to be concerned every day that you go to*
> *work that something may happen.*

Some people may scoff at the notion that these assaults are enough to change a life. Yet consider one veteran emergency room nurse who's patient strangled her with a stethoscope. The outcome of her experience? She suffered physical injuries and emotional trauma, she received very little support from her director, and she decided to leave nursing entirely after more than two decades as an ER nurse.

> *I left the job I loved and knew. I just don't want to get hurt*
> *again.*

# TRUE ACCOUNTS

There are countless examples of healthcare violence; the following are just a handful.

From *I Am Fine but Violence in the ED is Not*[14]:

> *The ED was at its worst, full to capacity, all healthcare personnel were stretched to the limit. I knew I needed to find a room and assess the patient quickly, complaints of chest pain and high blood pressure are very serious. The man was put on a stretcher and wheeled into a room, I was putting on the blood pressure cuff, oxygen monitor and cardiac leads. The patient was demanding to call his wife, I explained to the patient that as soon as I was able to take his blood pressure he could call his wife. I knew this patient from another hospital admission when I had taken care of him every day. I tried to calm him and started to say something when all of a sudden the patient punched me. He punched me so hard in my face that the force of that punch moved my body against a cart that holds our supplies...*

---

[14] Originally published on www.nursing.advanceweb.com.

From *Danger zone: Workplace violence touches many in nursing*[15]:

*Paula, a 50-year-old healthcare worker, was kicked multiple times in the upper body by a 24-year-old patient. She described how the attack affected not only her but her 4-year-old grandson:*

*"This isn't the first time I have been assaulted, but the saddest thing was when my 4-year-old grandson saw my bruises. He was frightened. I couldn't imagine telling him that a patient hurt me, so I lied and said I fell! The look on his face was enough to make me cry…he said to me, 'Grandma you are really hurt! I went to hug him and as I looked at him he was crying…The patient who kicked me has hurt not only me, but my whole family. I could just scream if I had the energy and I wasn't in so much pain…I get so angry thinking that a young man thinks it is all right to kick someone the way he kicked me and not care."*

§

## But Wait, There's More

Boston Brigham and Women's surgeon Michael Davidson was shot and killed in January 2015 by the son of a deceased patient.

§

---

[15] www.tinyurl.com/nurse-danger-zone

Jeaux Rinehart, a registered nurse for more than 30 years, was working at Virginia Mason Medical Center in 2008 when a patient seeking methadone attacked him with a billy club, breaking his cheekbone.

A 68-year-old Minnesota hospital patient, Charles Emmett Logan, violently attacked hospital staff with a metal bar in November 2014, injuring four nurses.

In June 2016 a Texas ER nurse was struck in the face with a clipboard at the hands of a patient.

An Oklahoma City nurse was sexually assaulted by a patient in October 2016.

So, yes: life can and does change in a heartbeat. In fact, Nurse.com[16] puts it very succinctly:

> *As healthcare workers, we never know whether we will return home in the same condition in which we started work - or even whether we will get home at all.*

---

[16] www.tinyurl.com/nurse-danger-zone

# BEYOND OUR BORDERS

## It's Everywhere

Healthcare violence is not limited to US-geographical boundaries. In fact, I have written a few articles[17] chronicling violent events against healthcare workers that have occurred outside of the United States.

In researching and writing on this topic, I have come to understand, with eye-opening horror, just how invasive healthcare violence has become.

It's not just happening here - in Massachusetts, New England, or even North America.

It is happening everywhere, and it is rampant.

These attacks have involved stabbings, concussions, broken bones, and even death at the hands of patients or patient family members.

---

[17] www.stophealthcareviolence.org/resources/articles-publications/

25

In April 2016, three UK-hospital nurses were viciously attacked by a patient's family member.

In May 2016, a UK psychiatric nurse was stabbed by a patient with a syringe.

Also in May 2016, a semi-retired London nurse tragically lost his life when he was attacked and stabbed by a patient.

In August 2016, a pregnant nurse working at Zhongnan Hospital in Wuhan, China, was punched in the face by a patient's son.

So it's clear: healthcare violence is not limited by geographical boundaries of Massachusetts, New England or even the United States, for that matter. It is happening everywhere.

And it needs to stop.

# VISIBLE - AND HIDDEN - DAMAGE

One of my nursing colleagues suffered a violent shove to the ground during a patient attack. She couldn't imagine why her shoulder hurt so badly afterward until she had an x-ray. The nurse had had hardware in her shoulder from a prior skiing accident, and the attack caused the hardware in her shoulder to became displaced. The resulting injuries required surgery and necessitated several months of missed work.

But the after-effects of her assault weren't limited to a shoulder injury and lost work. She was also afflicted with severe emotional distress.

## Post-Traumatic Stress Disorder

Beyond physical damage from workplace assault lies another aftermath: emotional trauma. Even if there are no physical injuries present, victims can become afflicted with anxiety, depression, and of course post-traumatic stress disorder, or PTSD. According to the Mayo Clinic[18]:

*Post-traumatic stress disorder (PTSD), is a mental health condition that's triggered by a terrifying event - either experiencing it or witnessing it. Symptoms may include*

---

[18] www.tinyurl.com/mayo-clinic-ptsd

*flashbacks, nightmares and severe anxiety, as well as uncontrollable thoughts about the event.*

Many people who experience traumatic events may have difficulty adjusting and coping for a while, but they don't necessarily develop PTSD. With time and good self-care, they recover. However, if post-trauma symptoms worsen, or last for months or even years and interfere with daily life functioning, the victim may have PTSD. Getting effective treatment after PTSD symptoms develop can be critical to reducing symptoms and improving function.

Often, incidents of healthcare violence and PTSD go hand-in-hand. Marcia, a triage nurse, described her symptoms:

*[The effects of the assault] hit me that night…I remember not being able to sleep…locking my doors, locking windows…*

And this, according to an abstract published by MedScape.com:

*In addition to physical injury, disability, chronic pain, and muscle tension, employees who experience violence suffer psychological problems such as loss of sleep, nightmares, and flashbacks…Health care workers who are assaulted experience shortterm and long-term emotional reactions, including anger, sadness, frustration, anxiety, irritability, apathy, self-blame, and helplessness…Symptoms occurred regardless of whether an injury was sustained from the assault.*

# THE RIPPLE EFFECT

Healthcare violence affects more than the victim. Like a ripple, these incidents bring about results and consequences that expand and spread outward incrementally.

Beyond impacting the victim, those waves can also rock friends and family, those witnessing the assault, colleagues, employers, and even consumers.

## Direct Impacts of Healthcare Violence

Healthcare violence directly affects…

- **the victim,** who suffers:
    - physical trauma or injuries
    - emotional distress such as PTSD
    - financial damage due to lost work days resulting from an event
- **the victim's friends, colleagues, and family, and those who hear or bear witness to the abuse.**

Ellen[19], a psychiatric nurse, echoes these principles:

*We have many, many people with PTSD, either from having witnessed the assault or having been assaulted themselves.*

## Indirect Impacts of Healthcare Violence

Healthcare violence indirectly affects…

- **the employer,** through:

    o staff shortages and its effects on colleagues and the public, due to injured employees who are unable to return to work immediately or full-time

    o financial repercussions - resulting from potential litigation and legal costs

- **you, the consumer and the community at large:**

    o employer costs will, inevitably, be passed on to you, the consumer

---

[19] www.tinyurl.com/youtube-4-victims

These concepts are plainly yet thoroughly outlined by The Online Journal of Nursing[20]:

*Major [direct] costs that result from acts of workplace violence are subsequent litigation from the party or parties involved...[with indirect costs] it is also very important to calculate lost work days that result from a violent event. The impact of lost wages on healthcare and nursing units may be seen indirectly in higher than average turnover; increased requests for medical leaves; unusually high time and attendance issues; and stress related illnesses.*

OSHA[21] further illustrates some of these impacts:

*Workplace violence comes at a high cost. If an employee requires medical treatment or misses work because of a workplace injury, workers' compensation insurance will typically have to pay the cost. For example, one hospital system had 30 nurses who required treatment for violent injuries in a particular year, at a total cost of $94,156 ($78,924 for treatment and $15,232 for lost wages). If your organization self-insures (as some large healthcare organizations do), it will bear the full cost. If your organization does not, its claim experience can still affect insurance premiums.*

---

[20] www.tinyurl.com/ana-wpv-in-healthcare
[21] www.tinyurl.com/osha-wpv-in-healthcare

Also according to OSHA, violence can also lead to other less obvious costs. For example:

- Caregiver fatigue, injury, and stress are tied to a higher risk of medication errors and patient infections.
- Studies have found higher patient satisfaction levels in hospitals where fewer nurses are dissatisfied or burned out.
- Injuries and stress are common factors that drive some caregivers to leave the profession. In 2013, the estimated cost of replacing a nurse is $27,000 to $103,000. This cost includes separation, recruiting, hiring, orientation, and training. Some estimates also account for lost productivity while a replacement is hired and trained.

# SILENT CONSENT AND OTHER CRAZINESS

## Why Is Healthcare Violence Escalating?

This question isn't easy. There are countless barriers interfering with curbing and stopping healthcare assaults and violence, and there are numerous government agencies and accredited industry organizations that have conducted studies on this same question. Let me see if I can tease some of it out from my perspective. But first, a reality check:

> *Recently workplace violence has gained recognition as a distinct category of violent crime that requires specific responses from employers, law enforcement and the community…*

This premise was quoted by the FBI *in 2004.*

As of this writing, it has been *12 years* since the FBI issued this premise, and the problem is worsening at an alarming rate. But, back to the question: why is healthcare violence escalating?

There is a myriad of elements and barriers that contribute to the persistence and worsening of healthcare violence, some of which is described by the APNA[22]:

*There are clinical, ethical, legal, and political dimensions to this occupational hazard that can serve as formidable barriers to prevention and harm reduction. Inurnment due to chronic and protracted exposure to violent individuals, underreporting, few effective external regulations, and the belief that violence is "just part of the job" are just a few of the roadblocks to effective violence prevention...*

*Nevertheless, barriers to effectively addressing the problem of workplace violence persist and include inconsistent legal and regulatory protections, widely varying prevention programs lacking an evidence base, the belief that violence is "part of the work," and the absence of standardized operational definitions precluding benchmarking and monitoring.*

So let's dive in and take a look at a few of these obstacles.

## The "It's-My-Job" Misconception

*"There is a top-to-bottom cultural assumption that violence is part of the job" for ER nurses and health-care workers, says Lisa Wolf, a registered nurse and research director for the Emergency Nurses Association. -Scientific American*[23]

---

[22] www.tinyurl.com/apna-position-statement
[23] www.tinyurl.com/n239vn4

The American Nurses Association[24] echoes:

> *The complexities [of workplace violence] arise, in part, from a health care culture resistant to the notion that health care providers are at risk for patient-related violence combined with complacency that violence (if it exists) "is part of the job."*

As does OSHA[25]:

> *Healthcare has some unique cultural factors that may contribute to underreporting or acceptance of workplace violence. For example, caregivers feel a professional and ethical duty to "do no harm" to patients. Some will put their own safety and health at risk to help a patient, and many in healthcare professions consider violence to be "part of the job." Healthcare workers also recognize that many injuries caused by patients are unintentional, and are therefore likely to accept them as routine or unavoidable. Another consideration is unwillingness among healthcare workers to stigmatize the perpetrators due to their illness or impairment.*

Dear reader, allow me to remind you: *No. Violence is not part of your job. No matter what.*

Federal law says so.

- Under federal law[26], you are entitled to a safe workplace. Your employer must provide a workplace free of known health and safety hazards.

---

[24] www.tinyurl.com/ana-wpv-in-healthcare
[25] www.tinyurl.com/osha-wpv-in-healthcare

Our professional organizations say so.

- The ENA[26] dictates that *emergency nurses have the right to personal safety in the work environment.*

- The ANA[28] states that *the nursing profession will no longer tolerate violence of any kind from any source.*

I say so, and so should you.

*It is not part of your job description to be violated or assaulted. If you believe that it is, please read that job description again.*

## The Blame Game

Has your nurse leader or administrator ever asked you, or a colleague, "What could you have done better to avoid the assault?"

I've witnessed this question being raised to healthcare coworkers, and it always flummoxed me. *Does this leader really believe the assault I or my colleague suffered was a result of something I did or did not do?*

I once confronted a manager with this exact response after she posed this question to one of my colleagues. When she responded with a look of confusion, I explained how ludicrous this question and its related thought process are. After our discussion, she realized the absurdity of the

---

[26] www.osha.gov/workers/index.html
[27] www.tinyurl.com/ena-position-statement
[28] www.tinyurl.com/ana-position-statement

question, and how its associated assumptions could negatively impact the assault victim. This may have been a teachable moment; as far as I know, she doesn't ask that anymore.

**Lack of Management Recognition, Commitment**

OSHA[29] identifies several risk factors when it comes to healthcare violence, including:

- Lack of facility policies and staff training for recognizing and managing escalating hostile and assaultive behaviors

- Lack of means of emergency communication

- Perception that violence is tolerated and victims will not be able to report the incident to police and/or press charges

In the same publication, OSHA states:

*Management commitment, including the endorsement and visible involvement of top management, provides the motivation and resources for workers and employers to deal effectively with workplace violence.*

Which begs the question, "So why isn't management on board with massive safety, training, and prevention programs?"

---

[29] www.tinyurl.com/osha-guidelines

Well, that leads to my next point:

**Looks are Everything**

Let me begin with three queries:

1. Does the administration really want us to report assaults?

2. Does the institution want a public record of employee assaults and subsequent involvement of law enforcement?

3. Does management want the community and the public at large to be aware of these occurrences of violent or unsafe incidents?

The simple answer to all: *of course not.*

It would make the institution look poorly and that clearly would not be good for business.

A healthcare assault victim feels as if she has virtually no rights.

Over 7,000 ER nurses completed an ENA questionnaire about Emergency Department (ED) violence.

Seventy-two percent of the respondents reported that the employing hospital had no response to episodes of physical abuse.

Eighty-one percent reported that the employing hospital had no response to complaints of verbal abuse.

That means that between roughly *three or four out of every five of your colleagues receive zero support from his or her employer.*

§

## What's Your Workplace Diagnosis?

Let me ask you: What's going on at your place of employment, and what is being done?

Do you observe any signage advocating against violence?

How many signs are visible and what do they say?

*Prominent signs using the word NO should be displayed throughout every facility, clearly describing behavior that is not tolerated.*

Are you or your colleagues holding or attending workplace violence meetings?

How often are such meetings held? Monthly? Annually?

Who is in attendance? Is staff invited? Do police personnel attend? Does anyone speak up or speak out?

When you, or a healthcare colleague, are assaulted, what happens? Is management supportive? Does someone assist the victim with an incident or police report? Is there any follow-up?

*After ER nurse Jane was violently pushed to the floor by a patient, she decided to end her shift and go home, handing her patients over to another nurse. Jane knew she should have stayed and completed an incident report about the assault; she knew she could have contacted the police and filed a report. These thoughts were present, but she simply couldn't handle what had happened.*[30]

Are medical charts flagged so that when a known violent perpetrator registers, hospital employees are immediately on alert that there is a history of aggressive behavior? Utilize an acuity tool that evaluates the risk of violence in order to determine if the patient meets the criteria.

Are you and your colleagues equipped with safety alarms or panic buttons? Do you have security staff manning the area at all times?

*…we always have a guard…whenever we see someone is [agitated or intoxicated] … the guards are inside the room with us, they stay there…but still, people can still hurt you… because sometimes they are so fast…you see a lot of problems…what we see a lot of here is family… that come with [the patient] who are more aggressive, sometimes, than the patient…but what we do, we have guards almost everywhere…we carry panic buttons…* Interview with Aruba ER nurse Ruben Croes[31]

---

[30] www.tinyurl.com/article-nurse-together
[31] www.tinyurl.com/youtube-interview-ruben

## Where Is The Coworker Who Cares?

Beyond the enormous need for employer support, there is a gaping need for colleague support. Very often there is no assistance or follow-up from management, and assault victims, already traumatized, are easily pushed aside without aid or advocacy; right at the critical time when colleague support can make a difference for the victim and how the incident is handled. Consider this scenario:

> *...I've been a nurse in the emergency department for 23 years. I worked with hundreds of patients and have been assaulted more times than I can count. This episode made me realize that when I asked for help it was being taken too lightly. The response from my coworkers and managers consisted of a shrug of the shoulder, eye roll, and 'I don't know what to tell you.' I knew the only way to keep myself safe was to end my career and move on...*[32]

After decades of working in the ER, this healthcare professional chose to end her nursing career. Asked what could have changed her mind about her decision to leave nursing, she said:

> *If only my coworkers would have listened to me and tried to understand what I was going through...We have all been assaulted and we all know what getting assaulted does to you. If the administration had come to me to ask, 'What can we do for*

---

[32] www.tinyurl.com/article-nurse-together

*you and to make this place safer?' I might have given it a second thought, but they didn't. Instead, I left a job I loved.*

Encouraging and fostering an environment of mutual colleague support begs the question, how do we train nurses and other staff to champion each other? It begins at the top. Read one of my last sections, What Employers Can Do, to probe this further.

# THE NEED FOR FELONY LEGISLATION

## Why Each State Must Pass and Enforce Laws with Stricter Penalties

As of this writing, there are 33 states[33] that have made assault on healthcare providers a felony.

That leaves 17 states that consider these assaults a misdemeanor.

*Meaning that almost two-thirds of all U.S. states have recognized the need for stricter laws and have passed felony-level statutes for healthcare worker assaults.*

And my home state of Massachusetts is *not* one of them.

### Felony vs Misdemeanor - What's the Difference?

What is the difference between a felony and misdemeanor?

First, let's look at an infraction: An infraction is similar to, say, being stopped by a police officer for driving over the speed limit. Usually, the penalty for this is a ticket – you are issued a citation to pay a fine, and you pay it.

---

[33] www.tinyurl.com/ena-state**s**

Next, there is a misdemeanor. A misdemeanor is more serious than an infraction. A misdemeanor means you could go to jail for up to a year - usually county jail, not prison – for committing a crime.

Lastly is a felony. Felonies are more serious crimes and jail time is usually greater than one year, with time served in a prison.

**Massachusetts: Failing to Pass**

As noted earlier, I live in Massachusetts, and Massachusetts is one of the 17 states that has failed to pass felony legislation.

In January 2015, I began lobbying extensively for the passage of Massachusetts House Bill 1164, which would do just that – increase penalties for assault on healthcare workers, changing it from a misdemeanor to a felony.

In March 2016, HB1164 failed to pass, and instead was sent to study – in other words, the Bill was tabled, stalled.

Shocked and astounded, I spoke with one Massachusetts legislative aide and asked why and how this could happen - after all, it seems to me that it's a no-brainer: *stiffer penalties equals more health worker protection which then translates into a reduction in violence.*

The aide told me that this Bill just didn't spark enough interest. I asked him what kind of bills *do* tend to get passed in the Massachusetts legislature.

The answer: liquor laws.

Which speaks volumes for Massachusetts State congressmen's priorities.

§

So now I am preparing for 2017 where I will tackle yet again the task of garnering support to pass Massachusetts legislation making assault on a healthcare worker a felony.

And I would encourage everyone reading this to do the same.

This is a new journey for me; I've never done this before. I have fought for many things, but going to the State House, speaking about the need for stiffer penalties, attending congressional functions, testifying to the Massachusetts Judiciary Committee - it's all new to me. It hasn't been easy and it hasn't always been fun. Yet in my humble opinion, we have no choice; it's a task that must be undertaken.

**What Difference Would it Make?**

Is it really so critical that we have laws treating these assaults as felonies, rather than misdemeanors? Will enacting stronger laws and enforcing stricter penalties *really* make a difference?

I don't have a crystal ball, but I know this much:

Assault on healthcare workers has become a crisis of epidemic proportions – one that is figuratively and literally screaming for more rigorous anti-assault laws. It's not simply me, or a handful of individuals, believing this to be true; *33 states - two-thirds of our nation* - have recognized this tenet and have answered the call for tougher laws by passing felony legislation; a position that is echoed by the Emergency Nurses Association[34]:

> *Violence in emergency departments has reached epidemic levels and emergency nurses are particularly vulnerable. In hopes of combating this violence in the emergency department, ENA believes that all states should make it a felony crime to commit assault and/or battery on an emergency nurse.*

So it all boils down to one simple concept:

*More stringent penalties mean more healthcare worker protection.*

**Tougher Laws Benefit All**

Tougher laws are sorely needed.

Tougher laws act as a deterrent, as a catalyst for more effective workplace violence and safety programs for our healthcare colleagues, and even as a means to garner help for the perpetrator.

Directly following the passage of felony legislation in the State of Utah[35], one ER nurse, ENA member, and assault victim reported on the outcome of her own experience pressing charges against her attacker under felony law:

---

[34] www.tinyurl.com/wpv-resources
[35] www.tinyurl.com/ena-praises-utah

*I thought you all should hear my assault news! She got 180 days in jail and two years' probation along with a mandatory drug program completion.*

And one more thing. As a human being, I hold a passionate position on this topic, and therefore I say this:

*It is just plain wrong to go to work with the risk that today just might be the day I, you, your son, daughter or friend, could be harmed and never able to return to work again due to a life-changing injury; an injury inflicted by someone who is not being held accountable for his or her actions or its consequences.*

PART II

# LET'S FIX THIS

## A STEP-BY-STEP REPAIR TOOLKIT

How do we fix the chaos of healthcare violence, and is it even possible?

The simple answer is: *yes.*

*We* can make it happen.

Read on for step-by-step means and methods that, working as individuals and working together, we can begin to harness this frightening and growing epidemic. Some steps are so simple as to seem inane, while others may appear more challenging. But everything is achievable.

Now, let's get to work.

## CHANGE YOUR MINDSET

First and foremost: change your mindset and way of thinking when it comes to healthcare violence if you haven't already.

**Don't Buy Into the Myths**

**MYTH: "It's part of my job."**

*No, no, no, no, no.*

It is not part of your job, and it is not within your job description.

Chances are, you or someone you know has heard colleagues say it is or implied that it is.

I don't care who says or thinks this; *it is not.*

Not only do you have the **right** to a safe workplace, **the law mandates it.**

OSHA law requires your workplace employer to **maintain the safety** of ALL healthcare workers.[36]

Further, the OSHA law also **prohibits employers from retaliating against employees** for exercising their rights under

---

[36] www.osha.gov/workers/index.html

the law, including the right to raise a health and safety concern or report an injury. Check out whistleblowers.gov or Workers' rights[37] under the OSH Act to learn more on government protection mandates.

And don't forget that our own industry professional organizations support us in this, as well. The ANA[38], the MNA[39], the Society of Trauma Nurses[40], and the American Psychiatric Nurses Association[41], among others, all publicly advocate for a safe workplace environment that must be fostered, established and maintained by organizational leadership.

Consider these Position Statement excerpted from said industry organizations:

> *The MNA believes that employers have a responsibility to provide safe and healthful working conditions in accordance with the Occupational Safety and Health Act of 1970. This includes preventing and addressing conditions that lead to violence and abuse and by implementing effective security and administrative work practices to protect the safety and health of workers.[42]*

---

[37] www.osha.gov/workers/index.html

[38] www.tinyurl.com/ana-position-statement

[39] www.tinyurl.com/mna-position-statement

[40] www.traumanurses.org/workplace-violence

[41] www.tinyurl.com/apna-position-statement

[42] www.tinyurl.com/mna-position-statement

*APNA supports a sustained commitment to fostering a safe and healthy workplace. APNA recognizes that the ultimate responsibility for maintaining the safety of staff and other individuals in treatment and learning environments rests with the nursing and administrative leadership of each setting.*[43]

*Statement of ANA Position:…the nursing profession will no longer tolerate violence of any kind from any source. All registered nurses and employers in all settings, including practice, academia, and research must collaborate to create a culture of respect, free of incivility, bullying, and workplace violence.*[44]

**MYTH: "It's not really that bad."**

It *is* that bad. The ENA states: Emergency nurses are at significant occupational risk for workplace violence.

In hospitals, nursing homes, and other healthcare settings, possible sources of violence include patients, visitors,

---

[43] www.tinyurl.com/apna-position-statement

[44] www.tinyurl.com/ana-position-statement

intruders, and even coworkers. Examples include verbal threats or physical attacks by patients, a distraught family member who may be abusive or even become an active shooter, gang violence in the emergency department, a domestic dispute that spills over into the workplace, or coworker bullying.

In a 2014 survey[45], almost 80 percent of nurses reported being attacked on the job within the past year. Health-care workers experience the most nonfatal workplace violence compared to other professions by a wide margin, with attacks on them accounting for almost 70 percent of all nonfatal workplace assaults causing days away from work in the U.S., according to data from the Bureau of Labor Statistics.

**MYTH: "It takes too long to complete an event report and besides, nothing changes!"**

First, allow me to acknowledge that after the trauma of an assault it is very difficult to concentrate on writing a report of any kind. My friends and colleagues: *this is why, in order to enact change, we cannot do this alone; we must all work together in mutual support as a team, just as we do in our daily jobs as healthcare professionals.*

---

[45] www.tinyurl.com/journal-emergency-nursing

**Ask and offer:** If you are the victim of an assault, *ask* for assistance from a colleague, someone who can document the incident while you are describing what happened, or otherwise support you however you need while you make a record of the incident. If you are the colleague, *offer* your assistance to the victim.

Second, I must allow that I, too, once felt that nothing would change, regardless of taking the time to complete an incident report. Well, guess what? *I discovered that we didn't make enough noise about it!* We completed the report, submitted it, and then…that was the end of it.

**Follow up:** My friends, *following up on the incident report is critical.* Not only are you confirming that your report was received, but you are reminding your administrators about the incident.

Third, and this is perhaps the most critical point: Under-reporting (i.e., failing to report) does not serve to sweep the assault under the rug; out of sight, out of mind. Conversely, failing to document and report the incident actually contributes to the violence.

**Failing to report - a chronic problem and a contributing factor:** It's a fact that underreporting is a chronic problem and leads to a multitude of negative results. According to the US National Library of Medicine National Institutes of Health[46]:

---

[46] www.tinyurl.com/under-reporting

*Underreporting hinders violence prevention efforts in two ways. First, underreporting results in an underestimation of the true extent of the problem, thus indicating less of a need for prevention of possible negative effects than may actually be warranted... Second, without knowledge of the full spectrum of violent events to which workers are exposed, prevention efforts can only be designed to affect limited aspects of the problem*

Remember, being assaulted is not in your job description, and *an incident report documenting the assault serves as the beginning of your paper trail and your protection.* It is documentation that you can bring to the police department, your physician, court, and anywhere else you think will help.

**So report, ask for and offer help in reporting if needed, and make noise!** And remember it isn't in any job description to get assaulted.

§

**MYTH: "My manager, coworkers and colleagues won't support me."**

A dear friend of mine recently described her 6-hour visit to a local emergency room. It had been a Saturday night and she described how the ER was extremely busy. What struck her was how seamlessly the staff worked together in mutual unity; asking, offering and receiving support; *a team.*

My colleagues, please remember this: in the healthcare setting, especially in an Emergency Room, we are all part of a team.

We cannot possibly do our job effectively if we don't work in tandem with mutual support. Backing a fellow teammate who has been assaulted is simply an extension of that. Certainly, there are those in any group who fail to work effectively with a group, but in the end, he or she loses. If we lead by example, like the Colleague Who Cares, and offer support, help, guidance, and encouragement just as we do every day in our healthcare jobs, we can work wonders.

# UTILIZE YOUR POWER

## The Power of Knowledge

Being armed with knowledge, awareness and information have never harmed anyone, and nothing has ever been achieved by sticking one's head in the sand. This is especially true when it comes to life's crises - and that's what healthcare violence is - a crisis.

Become informed; get educated and stay up-to-date on the topic, including recommended policies, preventive methods, laws, and legislation.

Learn how to recognize, avoid, or diffuse potentially violent situations by attending personal safety training programs.

Alert supervisors to any concerns about safety or security and report all incidents immediately in writing, and keep a copy.

Arm yourself with as much information as you can about healthcare violence.

The Online Journal of Nursing[47] furthers this recommendation:

---

[47] www.tinyurl.com/ana-wpv-strategies

*Ensuring that healthcare providers have the appropriate education and training to recognize, diffuse, and deescalate violent behaviors is essential.*

## How and Where?

Well, by reading this book you've already begun that process! But there's so much more.

The Resources section of this book is a great way to dive further into the topic of healthcare violence.

Peruse the Stop Healthcare Violence website[48], including the links and resources.

Contact Stop Healthcare Violence and take advantage of our services. Here's a list of some of the functions we offer:

- Education and outreach for individuals, groups, and organizations

- Assistance and guidance in the process of filing criminal charges

- Lobbying efforts for legislative change

Read as much as you can, talk to as many people as you can, contact as many organizations as you can, enroll in and attend educational conferences and seminars, and immerse yourself in the topic.

---

[48] www.stophealthcareviolence.org

# ADOPT YOUR OWN ZERO TOLERANCE POLICY

Advocates for mitigating healthcare violence are strongly supportive of a zero tolerance policy on an organizational level. So doesn't it also make sense that you adopt your own no-tolerance approach to healthcare violence on an individual level?

> *The mitigation of WPV requires a "zero tolerance" environment instituted and supported by hospital leadership. -ENA*[49]

> *One of the best protections employers can offer their workers is to establish a zero-tolerance policy toward workplace violence. -* OSHA[50]

Reject any direct or indirect message that you are to blame, you are responsible, or that it is part of your job.

*Don't accept workplace violence. Challenge any laissez-faire or dismissive attitude about it. And don't let it go unreported or undocumented.*

---

[49] www.tinyurl.com/ena-position-statement
[50] www.tinyurl.com/osha-wpv-fact-sheet

# BE A PROPONENT OF PREVENTION

## The Implementation of Prevention Programs: A Key to Success

*Lack of a violence prevention program is associated with an increased assault risk in hospitals. Health care organizations should implement an interdisciplinary approach to establish a workplace violence prevention program. Emergency nurses should play an integral role in all aspects of violence prevention planning and monitoring. Prevention strategies for reducing exposure to violence risk should include environmental designs to provide a safe workplace, administrative controls to ensure safe staffing patterns and adequate security measures, and training workers to recognize and manage potential assaults…Health care organizations should provide safety training programs specific to the emergency setting for health care workers to recognize, mitigate, avoid, and defuse potential violent situations. -ENA[51]*

*The MNA recommends that all healthcare employers implement a Workplace Violence Prevention Program that is consistent*

---

[51]www.ena.org/government/State/Documents/ENAWorkplaceViolencePS.pdf

*with OSHA* Guidelines for Preventing Workplace Violence to Health Care and Social Service Workers. -MNA[52]

This means:

- An established and documented workplace violence prevention program, with ongoing staff training and education.

- The program should also be incorporated into an employee handbook or manual of standard operating procedures.

- A mandate that the employer promptly investigate and follow up on all claims of workplace violence.

- Safety education and training for you, the employee: knowing what conduct is not acceptable, what to do if you witness or are subjected to workplace violence, and how to protect yourself.

- Clear guidelines for the reporting process - how to report an incident, to whom, and how to follow up.

OSHA[53] describes a successful Violence Prevention Program as follows:

*Violence Prevention Programs: A written program for workplace violence prevention, incorporated into an*

---

[52] www.tinyurl.com/mna-position-statement

[53] www.tinyurl.com/osha-guidelines

*organization's overall safety and health program, offers an effective approach to reduce or eliminate the risk of violence in the workplace. The building blocks for developing an effective workplace violence prevention program include:*

*(1) Management commitment and employee participation,*

*(2) Worksite analysis,*

*(3) Hazard prevention and control,*

*(4) Safety and health training, and*

*(5) Recordkeeping and program evaluation.*

*A violence prevention program focuses on developing processes and procedures appropriate for the workplace in question.*

Take a look at OSHA's Fact Sheet on Workplace Violence[54] as well as its Workplace Violence Prevention guidelines[55] that describe preventative components in more detail.

---

[54] www.tinyurl.com/osha-wpv-fact-sheet

[55] www.tinyurl.com/osha-wpv-prevention-guidelines

# TAKE TEN

If you take away anything from this book, I hope they are:

- the premise that *violence is not part of your job,* and

- *the ten steps to implement in the event of an attack.*

The following is from the MNA's **Ten Actions a Nurse Should Take if Assaulted at Work**[56]:

1. Get help. Get to a safe area.

2. Call 911 for police assistance, (it is your civil right to call the police).

3. Get relieved of your assignment.

4. Get medical attention.

5. Report the assault to your supervisor and union.

6. Get counseling or assistance for Critical Incident Stress Debriefing (CISD) to address concerns related to Post Traumatic Stress Disorder (PTSD).

7. Exercise your civil rights, file charges with the police.

---

[56] www.tinyurl.com/mna-take-10

8. Get copies of all reports and keep a diary of events.

9. Take photographs of your injuries.

10. Return to work only when you feel safe and supported

# THE FOUR R'S

It's critical that we understand and utilize The Four Rs Tool for healthcare violence:

- **Recognize:** How do I recognize an escalating patient or family?

- **Respond:** How do I respond to an escalating patient?

- **Report:** How should I document the incident when I file a report?

- **Reboot:** What do I do next?

Below are the answers to those questions in the simplest form. Additional detailed information can be found here: www.tinyurl.com/teresa-brunt-rn

**Recognize** these symptoms of an escalating patient:

- Angry

- Inappropriate laughter

- Fear

- Confusion

- Anxious

- Crying

- Restlessness

- Nervousness

- No eye contact

**Respond** by alerting the designated response team. Do not approach the patient without a designated buddy. Do not block access to an exit. At this point, an incident report should be created no matter the outcome.

- Remain calm

- Trust your instincts

- Do not try to reason with the patient or family member

- Encourage cooperation

**Report:** Event reports need to be simple but concise, and completed prior to going home after an incident occurs. This document should stand as your accurate account of an incident.

**Reboot and debrief:** Talk about it! What could have been differently? Support for staff involved is crucial.

# TALK IT OUT

Don't keep this topic in the closet. Talk with colleagues about healthcare violence.

I and my colleagues are on the same team; and as a team, we need discussion and dialog.

Ask your nursing friends and colleagues:

- Have you ever been assaulted?

- What did you do about it?

- Did you complete incident reports, file police reports, press charges?

- Did you bring the perpetrator to court?

Be vocal and send the message to your healthcare colleagues: *tolerating assault is wrong. Don't accept it.*

Advocate for a culture of safety and support for a comprehensive violence prevention program.

Participate in interactive education programs about workplace violence and its prevention.

Share, and encourage coworkers to share, information about ways to avoid potentially violent situations.

Seek to empower registered nurses to respond appropriately to real or perceived violent situations.

If your facility does not have a workplace violence safety committee, policy or program, discuss your concerns with your peers and make sure your facility implements an effective violence prevention program.

Starting a dialogue, bringing the topic of healthcare violence out into the open, raising awareness, and vocalizing the mandate for a safe and secure environment are crucial elements in halting this epidemic, saving careers, preserving emotional stability, and even preserving a life.

## SUPPORT YOUR PEERS

As I've implied earlier, nursing is a team sport!

When it comes to healthcare violence, there are so many things, large and small, that we can do to support our colleagues. These are just a few:

- Encourage your colleague to report and log any incident or threat of violence, both with the institution as well as the police.

- Offer support in completing an incident report or filing a police report. Offer to write/document the incident report while your colleague describes the event; offer to accompany him or her on a police interview.

- Encourage your colleague to get prompt medical evaluation and treatment after an incident. Offer to accompany him or her if needed.

- Encourage your colleague to understand the right to report and prosecute the perpetrator.

- Support your colleague's need to seek EAP assistance, counseling or therapy if required.

- Advocate for yourself and your colleagues by vocalizing the need for WPV prevention programs and employee support.

# REPORT, REPORT, REPORT!

## First: How and Why Reporting is So Critical

Before I cover the aspect and process of reporting violent events to employers, law enforcement, and other officials, it's important to understand just how crucial reporting is to curbing healthcare violence, and how a breakdown in reporting contributes to the ongoing epidemic.

## Failing to Report: A Barrier to Improvement

Reporting violent events to employers as well as law enforcement and other officials is absolutely critical to curbing this epidemic.

It bears repeating and expanding upon this principle by quoting from the US National Library of Medicine National Institutes of Health[57]:

*Underreporting of violent events has been defined as failure of victimized employees to report these events to their employers,*

---

[57] www.tinyurl.com/under-reporting

*the police, or other officials… **Underreporting hinders
violence prevention efforts in two ways.** First,
underreporting results in an underestimation of the true extent
of the problem, thus indicating less of a need for prevention of
possible negative effects than may actually be warranted…
Second, without knowledge of the full spectrum of violent events
to which workers are exposed, prevention efforts can only be
designed to affect limited aspects of the problem…*

*Incident reports documenting adverse events can be used to
calculate incidence and prevalence rates, identify risk factors,
and develop prevention efforts for specific occupational hazards.
However, **underreporting of adverse workplace events is a
significant barrier to injury prevention** generally, and to the
prevention of workplace violence (WPV) specifically. In the
health care industry, WPV poses one of the most serious threats
to worker health and safety, **but underreporting has long been
a recognized barrier to improvement.***

In a nutshell:

- Underreporting has been a chronic problem

- Reporting all threats, assaults, stalking, and harassment
  must be consistent to bring public attention to this
  problem

- Violent acts should be a part of public record no matter
  where they occur.

- Reporting may serve as a deterrent if prosecution becomes a routine consequence of violent behavior.

## Why the Breakdown?

So why is there such a failure in the reporting process? Again quoting from the US National Library of Medicine[58]:

> *In health care, various reasons for underreporting WPV have included lack of injury or time lost, time-consuming incident reporting procedures, lack of supervisory or coworker support, fear of reprisal or blame, belief that reporting will not lead to any positive changes, and the common perception among health care workers that violence is simply "part of the job". Varying definitions of violence among employees and within organizations can also affect reporting behavior.*

So while it's no wonder we've been failing to report violent events, it's paramount that my colleagues in healthcare understand this breakdown needs to change. Read on for how to do that (information and guidelines courtesy of Susan Vickory, RN, C).

## Reporting To Your Employer

These are critical guidelines to follow in the event of an episode of healthcare violence:

---

[58] www.tinyurl.com/under-reporting

**First things first...**

- Call the Nursing Supervisor

- Call Hospital/Campus Police or Security Service to complete a Campus Police/Security Report

**The Incident Report...**

- Complete an Incident Report

- Document JUST THE FACTS

- Include time and date and who was notified

- Provide an objective description of the event; use specific and accurate statements

- Include a patient assessment and/or comments made by the patient or perpetrator

- Exclude any personal opinions or vague statements

- Any reference to an incident report

- Respond in a cautious manner to any question that may imply blame, such as "What could you have done to prevent this?"

- Ask a colleague to assist you in this process, if need be

## Physical Assessment, Documentation...

- Go to the Emergency Room or Employee Health Service

- Take photos of any injuries

- Save copies of all reports, photos, and documentation for your personal records.

- Keep a diary.

## Reporting To Law Enforcement

## Filing Criminal Charges...

While it may seem daunting, the filing of criminal charges is something that will protect and empower you, and also serve to protect others in the same situation.

- File a Police Report within five days

- Charges may be filed directly at District Court

- Hospital Police may file for the injured party

Ask a friend or colleague to assist you in this process, if need be

## The Legal Process...

- You will receive notification of a date for a hearing by mail.

- IMPORTANT: If your hearing is with a Court Magistrate, this will determine if your case will go to a judge for arraignment

- Prepare a written statement about what happened and what you would like to see happen. You may include how this has affected you both physically and psychologically.

- Bring witnesses or co-workers who can confirm your story

- Bring pictures of your injuries, medical reports, and the police or security report

- Once your case goes to a judge, an Assistant District Attorney (the prosecutor) will handle your case. You don't need to hire a lawyer.

- Victim Witness Advocate will meet with you and witnesses to explain the court procedures

- The Assistant District Attorney will keep you informed as to dates of court appearances

- The defendant will be referred to the Court Clinic for evaluation if competency or mental illness is an issue. If this happens, inform the Assistant District Attorney that you would like to speak with the evaluator.

- Submit a victim impact statement

## The Trial...

- The defendant will have the right to choose between a trial by jury or a trial by the judge

- The Assistant District Attorney will prepare you, the victim, and witnesses for testimony

- You will have the right to speak in court in front of the judge

### One Victim Speaks

As one ER nurse attested after filing criminal charges against her attacker:

*I thought you all should hear my assault news! She got 180 days in jail and two years' probation along with a mandatory drug program completion.* **If you ever question pressing charges, DO IT!** *Let's not let these people get away with beating us up.*

### Stop Healthcare Violence: Here to Help

It's important to note that Stop Healthcare Violence is available to guide you through the legal process. We are just a phone call or email away[59].

---

[59] www.stophealthcareviolence.org

## PART III

# EMPLOYER RESPONSIBILITY

## WHAT CAN YOUR EMPLOYER OR ADMINISTRATOR DO?

# WHAT EMPLOYERS AND ADMINISTRATORS CAN (AND SHOULD) DO

Industry organizations such as OSHA have long advocated for specific steps to be taken by employers to help protect their employees.

## Zero Tolerance

OSHA, as well as state and national healthcare agencies, advocate that the best protection employers can offer is to establish a zero-tolerance policy toward workplace violence against or by their employees.

Which then begs the question, how does this zero tolerance policy manifest itself?

## A Comprehensive Prevention Program

OSHA[60] advocates that employers establish and maintain a comprehensive, written violence prevention program as part of their facility's safety and health program:

---

[60] www.tinyurl.com/osha-wpv-in-healthcare

*Healthcare facilities can reduce workplace violence by following a comprehensive workplace violence prevention program. An effective program includes five key components:*

- *Management commitment and worker participation*

- *Safety and health training*

- *Worksite analysis and hazard identification*

- *Recordkeeping and program evaluation*

- *Hazard prevention and control*

OSHA[61] recommends that the prevention program should be made available to all employees, including managers and supervisors; and all employees should receive specific training concerning its content and implementation. The program should also track progress in reducing work-related assaults.

OSHA advocates that the main components of a Violence Prevention Program be:

- Management commitment and employee Involvement

- Demonstrated concern for employee emotional and physical safety, health, and security

- Worksite Analysis: A step by step common sense examination of the workplace to identify existing or potential hazards for workplace violence

---

[61] www.tinyurl.com/osha-wpv-hazards

- Safety and Health Training: To make all staff aware of security hazards and how to protect themselves through established policies, procedures, and training

- Recordkeeping and evaluation of the program

And from the APNA:

*APNA recognizes that the ultimate responsibility for maintaining the safety of staff and other individuals in treatment and learning environments rests with the nursing and administrative leadership of each setting.*

**Employer Support for Staff**

However, a comprehensive prevention program does nothing if it lacks consistent and thorough employee training and support.

OSHA points out that it is critical to ensure that all employees know the prevention program and policies, and understand that all claims of workplace violence will be investigated and remedied promptly.

Much more information on employer safety recommendations may be found in the Resources section of this book.

---

[62] www.tinyurl.com/apna-position-statement

[63] www.tinyurl.com/osha-wpv-fact-sheet

PART IV

# RESOURCES

## AFL-CIO NOW

- Workplace Violence: Not Part of the Job
  https://aflcio.org/2016/6/2/workplace-violence-not-part-job

## AMERICAN NURSES ASSOCIATION (ANA)

- ANA website
  http://nursingworld.org

- Position Statement
  http://www.nursingworld.org/MainMenuCategories/Workpl
  aceSafety/Healthy-
  Nurse/bullyingworkplaceviolence/Incivility-Bullying-and-
  Workplace-Violence.html

## CENTERS FOR DISEASE CONTROL AND PREVENTION (CDC)

- Occupational Violence
  https://www.cdc.gov/niosh/topics/violence/

# EMERGENCY NURSES ASSOCIATION (ENA)

- Emergency Department Violence Surveillance Study
  https://www.ena.org/practice-
  research/research/Documents/ENAEDVSReportNovember2
  011.pdf

- Hot Topics: Workplace Violence:
  https://www.ena.org/about/media/Pages/Hot-Topics.aspx

- Position Statement
  https://www.ena.org/government/State/Documents/ENAW
  orkplaceViolencePS.pdf

- ENA Praises Utah for Increased Workplace Protection
  https://finance.yahoo.com/news/emergency-nurses-
  association-praises-utah-140000103.html

- State Laws
  https://www.ena.org/government/State/Pages/Default.aspx

- Workplace Violence Toolkit
  https://www.ena.org/practice-
  research/Practice/ToolKits/ViolenceToolKit/Documents/tool
  kitpg1.htm

- Workplace Violence Resources
  https://www.ena.org/government/State/Pages/WVResourc
  es.aspx

## JOURNAL OF EMERGENCY NURSING

- Incidence and Cost of Nurse Workplace Violence Perpetrated by Hospital Patients or Patient Visitors http://www.sciencedirect.com/science/article/pii/S0099176 71300216X

## MASSACHUSETTS NURSES ASSOCIATION (MNA)

- MNA website http://www.massnurses.org

- Workplace Violence and Abuse Prevention and Position Statement http://www.massnurses.org/nursing-resources/position-statements/workplace-violence

- Workplace Violence: Ten Actions a Nurse Should Take If Assaulted at Work http://www.massnurses.org/health-and-safety/current-topics/workplace-violence/10-actions

## MAYO CLINIC

- PTSD http://www.mayoclinic.org/diseases-conditions/post-traumatic-stress-disorder/home/ovc-20308548

## ONLINE JOURNAL OF ISSUES IN NURSING

- Workplace Violence in Healthcare: Recognized but Not Regulated
http://nursingworld.org/MainMenuCategories/ANAMarketp lace/ANAPeriodicals/OJIN/TableofContents/Volume92004/N o3Sept04/ViolenceinHealthCare.html

- Workplace Violence in Healthcare: Strategies for Advocacy
http://nursingworld.org/MainMenuCategories/ANAMarketp lace/ANAPeriodicals/OJIN/TableofContents/Vol-18-2013/No1-Jan-2013/Workplace-Violence-Strategies-for-Advocacy.html

## OSHA/US DEPARTMENT OF OCCUPATIONAL SAFETY AND HEALTH ADMINISTRATION

- Caring for our Caregivers: Preventing Workplace Violence
https://www.osha.gov/Publications/OSHA3827.pdf

- Guidelines for Preventing Workplace Violence
https://www.osha.gov/Publications/osha3148.pdf

- Recommendations: Conducting a Workplace Security Analysis
https://www.ena.org/practice-research/Practice/ToolKits/ViolenceToolKit/Documents/OSH A%20analysis.htm

- The Whistleblower Protection Programs
https://www.whistleblowers.gov

- Worker Safety
  https://www.osha.gov/workers/index.html

- Worker Safety in Hospitals
  https://www.osha.gov/dsg/hospitals/workplace_violence.ht
  ml

- Workplace Violence
  https://www.osha.gov/SLTC/workplaceviolence/

- Workplace Violence Fact Sheet
  https://www.osha.gov/OshDoc/data_General_Facts/factshe
  et-workplace-violence.pdf

- Workplace Violence in Healthcare - Understanding the
  Challenges
  https://www.osha.gov/Publications/OSHA3826.pdf

- Workplace Violence Prevention guidelines
  https://www.osha.gov/SLTC/etools/hospital/hazards/workpl
  aceviolence/viol.html

## ROBERT WOOD JOHNSON FOUNDATION

- Nurses Face Epidemic Levels of Violence at Work
  http://www.rwjf.org/en/library/articles-and-
  news/2015/07/nurses-face-epidemic-levels-of-violence-at-
  work.html

## SCIENTIFIC AMERICAN

- Epidemic of Violence Against Health Care Workers Plague Hospitals
  https://www.scientificamerican.com/article/epidemic-of-violence-against-health-care-workers-plagues-hospitals/

## STOP HEALTHCARE VIOLENCE (SHCV)

- SHcV website
  http://stophealthcareviolence.org

- Contact/Inquiries
  http://stophealthcareviolence.org/inquiries/

- Links and Resources
  http://stophealthcareviolence.org/resources/links-resources/

- Our Services
  http://stophealthcareviolence.org/our-services/

- YouTube channel
  https://www.youtube.com/user/stophealthcareviolen

## US NATIONAL LIBRARY OF MEDICINE NATIONAL INSTITUTES OF HEALTH

- Underreporting of Workplace Violence
  https://www.ncbi.nlm.nih.gov/pmc/articles/PMC5006066/

## US DEPARTMENT OF LABOR (DOL)

- Healthcare Wide Hazards - Workplace Violence, Violence Prevention Plan
  https://www.osha.gov/SLTC/etools/hospital/hazards/workplaceviolence/viol.html

## OTHER

- American Psychiatric Nurses Association: Workplace Violence Position Statement
  http://www.apna.org/files/public/APNA_Workplace_Violence_Position_Paper.pdf

- Society of Trauma Nurses: Position Paper: Workplace Violence
  http://www.traumanurses.org/workplace-violence

- The 4 Rs Tool: Recognize, Respond, Report, Reboot
  http://avtbrunt.wixsite.com/teresabrunt/the-4r-s-tool

# ACKNOWLEDGMENTS

This book would not have been possible without the generous assistance of many. I am eternally grateful to my two wonderful nursing colleagues, Elizabeth McTomney, RN, and Sheryl Williams, RN, BSN. Together the three of us co-founded Stop Healthcare Violence, launching what has become an awesome and inspiring whirlwind of a journey. I have the utmost respect for, and gratitude toward, Teresa Brunt, RN, BSN, CSN, who was instrumental in passing Utah felony legislation (the 33rd state!) and who has selflessly shared her knowledge and experiences with me. A great portion of this book would be incomplete without the collaboration of Susan Vickory, RN, C, with her expertise in incident reporting, filing criminal charges, and the legal process. To my graphic designer and editor, Jamie Lyn Ross of Fat Cat Design; I love you, girl! To my friend and Board member, Jeanne White, who has made endless trips with me to the Massachusetts State House, and kept me sane over coffee at Panera. And to the countless others who have been by my side, literally and figuratively, for eight-plus years now, and counting - thank you; you all rock.

# ABOUT THE AUTHOR

Sheila Wilson, RN, BSN, MPH, is an emergency room nurse, leader, and activist. She has worked both in clinical and administrative management positions, as well as executive leadership roles. As a clinician and in-patient care manager, she works with HIV/AIDS, TB, and substance abuse patients, as well as under-served populations in the Boston area. Sheila conducts ongoing educational training and outreach services on a multitude of topics including her latest endeavor, workplace violence, and has been published in a number of print and online magazines and journals. She enjoys spending her free time surrounded by friends, colleagues, her husband, children, and grandchildren.

*For more information*

www.stophealthcareviolence.org
info@stophealthcareviolence.org